How Cancer Saved My Life

I Will Not Shed Another Tear

by

Y. Althea Boyer

M. Ed.

authorHOUSE®

AuthorHouse™
1663 Liberty Drive, Suite 200
Bloomington, IN 47403
www.authorhouse.com
Phone: 1-800-839-8640

First published by AuthorHouse   6/12/2008

ISBN: 978-1-4343-7662-6 (sc)

Library of Congress Control Number: 2008905164

Printed in the United States of America
Bloomington, Indiana

This book is printed on acid-free paper.

Cover Design by Akemi Carter

Table of Contents

Dedication

Honey,

I could not have written this book without your continuous support and undying love for me throughout this whole ordeal. When you asked me to marry you, I'm sure you didn't anticipate cancer would soon join our happy life. When it did come uninvited, you didn't run for the nearest exit, or into the arms of another woman, but you stood by me and fought this battle with me, side by side, and for this, I am truly blessed and forever grateful.

You are what a real man is supposed to be. You stood firm when everything came crashing down around us, and you continued to look upward, waiting and expecting God to move. You knew when to push me and when to simply step back and let me have my own way because you knew that was what I needed at that moment. You allowed me to find my own way without controlling or hindering me.

No one knows the sacrifices you made for us but you and God. I know a little, but I'm sure I don't know the whole story, because you always kept that away from me, instead encouraging me to focus on my health and to find my way to God.

My heart aches for all the pain this disease caused you and caused our family, but I thank you for always being here regardless. You never left. Even when I tried to push you away to spare you this grief, you never left.

Honey, when we prayed together, you'd always ask God for restoration and to make the devil pay back what he has stolen from us. God heard your prayers, and He will replace and restore double what the enemy has stolen from us. The Lord says, "I will restore unto you the years that the locust hath eaten, the cankerworm, and the caterpillar, and the palmerworm" (Joel 2:25).

When I wasn't strong enough, you had strength for both of us. Thank you for standing beside me throughout all of this. The best is yet to come. This I decree and declare! Now, let's walk into the restoration together.

Thank you, baby and I love you!

Acknowledgements

Miyako (my hero): Thank you for making good choices all these years. I didn't have to worry about what you were doing, and that made it so much easier for me to focus on my health. I'm sorry I wasn't the mother I wanted to be because I was always sick, but you are turning into such a beautiful young woman. Now, you are in college, and God allowed me to be here to see it. I am so proud of you. Keep God close to you, baby. He is the only way. I love you. *Life has not been easy for you, but I see you at a place of complete peace in your life. You will have the desires of your heart, but God must be in the midst, for your dreams are in <u>His</u> hands.*

Teruko: Thank you for the phone calls, cards, and beautiful letters you wrote. They always came just when I needed them most. Things happened for a reason, but I am glad we are here now. God has always had His Hand over you. Listen to Him. He has so much in store for you. I love you. *Your life has been very hard, but I see easier times ahead for you. All of your dreams are within your grasp, but the key is God. The sooner you realize that He is the way, the sooner He will release the blessings He has stored up for* *you. I see them raining on you. Press your way to Him. He's waiting.*

My sisters: Once we laughed for twenty minutes because you had both gone to church and forgotten to pray for me. Thank you for that, because it showed me the awesome faith you had in God. You already were where I was striving to be. Your love and support mean the world to me. You are the best sisters in the world.

Miko: There is a peace and serenity about you that is so beautiful. You really have found that place in God that most people only dream of. Nothing seems to shake you. Even when things do go "crazy", most people's initial response is to "freak out", but you simply seek God and wait on Him to answer. When I think of the perfect family, wife and mother, I think of you. Your deep desire to minister to the family is evident in your ability to lovingly and tenderly minister to your own family. Corey is a blessed man! Thank you for forcing me to dig deeper to finish this book. *I see you ministering to families, and many marriages will be saved because you led them to God's way. You've had to go through much because you will help many.*

Aki: You are the wild flower in the family. No matter what life throws at you, you continue to thrive with beauty and grace. You have a child like faith in God that we should all seek to have. God has given you creativity, an eye to see beauty in everything, and a love for people that is unreal. Your ability to easily forgive and love others "in spite of" continues to astound me. I love you and thank you for designing my book cover. It is breath-taking! It means more to me than you can ever imagine. *I see many doors opening up for you because you have remained so faithful to Him. A new beginning is on the way for you, but not in the way you expect.*

Echi: You have the grit and tenacity that will take you far. I will always remember that first Thanksgiving we all spent together in Vegas. You will never know how special that moment was for me. It is forever etched into my heart. Mama and Daddy would be so proud of the man you have become. I love you! *You have a sharp business mind and a very unique way of relating to people. Something about you draws people towards you. God is going to use those attributes for His glory. Get ready!*

Mrs B.: Thank you for all your heartfelt prayers. You seemed to always know just when to bring some good food over. It was always at just the right time. I really do appreciate it! Love ya!

Pastors: You have been there for me by praying, calling, giving me books to read, encouraging me, and not letting go of me in the spirit. As busy as you both are, you always have time to talk to me. You make me feel like my trials are the most important thing to you, and I love you both for that. I have grown so much under your ministry. You both truly have the heart and love of a servant of God. I will be forever grateful to both of you for all you have done for me.

Karen: You are the trailblazer, and the "breaker" anointing is on you.   Your life has been hard because He was preparing you for such a time as this.   He will use you to break down barriers.   I am watching and learning so much from you. Thank you for all your help and prayers. *This is only the beginning for you.   You carry a heavy load because there is much work you have to do in His kingdom.   There are places God is going to take you that even you have not "seen".*

Debbie: You have been there praying and watching out for me. You've always "had my back" and I can't begin to thank you enough.   You knew how important it was for me to walk through this thing privately, and you respected that. I remember you telling me years ago, to do whatever I had to do, however I had to, but to just get through it.   Thank you for always being there.

Pamelia: Your grace and walk with God is unquestionable. Throughout your own trials, you still reach out to other women through the organization you founded, *Women of Destiny*.   You continuously put yourself aside to minister to the needs of other people.   Pam, you are such a dedicated servant of God.   Thank you for all your insight, wisdom, and prayers.   You are a true woman of God.

Peggy: You have always been able to "read" me.   You knew when I wasn't feeling well no matter how much I tried to hide it, and you'd just help me, even when I didn't realize that I needed it. You are such a dear friend. Thank you for all your help, continuous support and prayers.

Brian and Allison: Thank you, thank you, and thank you. It would have been so much harder if it wasn't for you. Thank you!

Jackie and Dan: Thank you for your prayers and for keeping my secret as I walked through this in my own way. It was such a blessing to know that I could talk to you openly and know that you would keep my secret as if it were your own. **Jackie**, thank you for…you know what!

Dr S.: I prayed that God would give me the best doctor and He gave you to me. This is so much more than a career to you. You are a brilliant woman with a big heart, and you genuinely care about people. You always made me feel like I was more than just a patient, but that I really mattered. You have fought this battle with me, side by side. That's why you are so successful and sought-after. I understand why people say you are the "best in the field." God bless you. It is a blessing and an honor to know you.

Her Staff: Thank you for treating me like family. It was hard enough just to go through everything, but you all made it so much easier by just being you. You are the best.

Larry and Steve: You both are best friends of my husband. Although he is a very private person, thank you for always being there for him, just in case he needed or wanted to talk.

All my family and friends: Thank you for your continuous prayers, phone calls to check up on me, our traditional Christmas dinners, and real friendship. It means the world to me.

Chapter One

The Beginning of a Nightmare

Who would have thought that I, of all people, would get cancer? I didn't smoke, drink, or even party. I was married to a wonderful man, and I had a real family, a nuclear family. I was a teacher and lived a good moral life, yet here I was diagnosed with that dreaded "C" word. That word that would change my life forever. That word that started me on a roller-coaster journey over which I had no control. That word that was sent to kill me.

It all started one beautiful summer day in August, 1996. I had only been teaching for two years. As a teacher, I had my summers off, and I was going to enjoy every moment of it. I had spent from June to the first week of August getting my lessons together, rewriting activities, and making up fun games for the coming new year. Life was finally going well. That is, it was finally going the way I thought it should be.

I began teaching in 1994 in a suburb. I was excited and wanted to be the best teacher I could be. I had many innovative ideas on how to make a difference in a child's life, but I especially wanted to help mold children to be loving and kind to others. I wanted to teach them to believe in themselves, and above all, I wanted to teach them that dreams can come to life if you only persevere.

Being a child of a bi-racial marriage, I faced many challenges growing up. English was my second language, but back then, they didn't have programs to support people like me. As a result, I was the girl who was put in a "slow" reading class throughout elementary school.

I went from someone who was thought of in elementary school as "retarded" to someone who stayed on the dean's list in college. I went from someone who was considered a "lost cause" to one who now holds a master's degree in education. Yes, I was always the underdog, but I wanted to show children that it's not how you start, but how you end that matters.

This was the thought that permeated my mind in that beautiful, perfect summer of 1996. I finally felt comfortable with teaching, and my family was wonderful. My husband had just surprised me with the best birthday present ever. He gave me the car of my dreams: a brand-new, bright red Mitsubishi 3000. I was on top of the world! What more could I want or need? Life was perfect. I was content and felt energized. I even started an exercise routine of lifting weights. Although I was a size 10/12, I wanted to tone up a little and knew that this would do the trick.

After about one month of working out, I noticed a crease in my right breast. It didn't really bother me, because I was right-handed and concluded that I was over-working my right muscle during my workouts, so I took a week off. Nothing changed. I took another week off, and still no change. I decided to get a checkup, and the appointment was made for the end of August, right before school started back after Labor Day. Perfect timing. I went early that morning to get my classroom ready and would stop by my doctor's office for this checkup and swing back to the classroom to finish up. The day went well until I arrived at my doctor's office. She was running behind schedule. After waiting forty-five minutes, I was told there were three other people ahead of me. I have never been a very patient person and kept thinking of all the things I could get accomplished in the classroom, so I made another appointment for October and left. I wasn't worried. After all, school was back in session, and I certainly wouldn't have time to work out anymore, and things would go back to normal.

September came and went, and then it was October. I went to the appointment as planned, but was a little annoyed because the crease hadn't gone away. My doctor, who is a female, examined me and said everything looked fine. She didn't understand the crease, but she didn't feel anything either during the exam. I kept questioning her about it, and she finally suggested a mammogram. Although I was too young for one, she said it would be a good idea to have a baseline on file, so I had a mammogram. The report came back as a suspicious growth, and a biopsy was scheduled. I went to a breast surgeon with the mammogram films in my hand. The doctor examined me, looked at the film, examined me again and said, "I agree. I think we need to do a biopsy. I don't feel anything at all, but I don't like the looks of this film. If it wasn't for this film, I would tell you there is nothing wrong and to go home, but this is why mammograms are so important."

My mind began to swirl around, and I felt sick to my stomach. *She is talking as if there might really be something wrong with me. Surely not. Not me. I'm one of the good people who likes to help other people out, and she is talking about a biopsy? What do I tell my husband? What about my family? No, this can't be. I just have to think positive, and everything will be fine.* People were always talking about the power of positive thinking, and now I would have to put that into practice...and so I did. I had the biopsy and went about my normal routine.

About four days later, I had just dropped my seven-year-old daughter off at a Brownie meeting and had just walked in the house when the phone rang. It was my doctor. There was something in her voice that didn't sound right, and then she said it: "I'm sorry, but the growth is cancerous. It was so deep in your muscle it couldn't be felt by a regular exam. Blah, blah, blah, blah, blah."

My legs gave out on me, and I slumped down on the couch. My whole body had gone ice-cold, and my hands were clammy as I gripped the phone. She said some other things to me during that conversation, but all I remember hearing was the word *cancerous.* I thanked her for calling, and I walked into the kitchen, where my husband was, and simply fell into his arms. All that positive thinking hadn't done anything. I had cancer. I was going to die.

My mind raced with questions, thoughts, and concerns. *Who will raise my daughter? I won't get to have that mother/daughter talk with her. I'll never see her finish school and go on to college. I won't*

4

see her married, and I'll never hold my grandchildren, just like Mom didn't. What about my husband? Who will take my place? Will he love her more? Will he gaze into her eyes like he does mine? How will she treat my daughter? Will they both forget about me? Will she raise her like I would have, with the same values and morals I hold dear?

God must have made a mistake! I knew women who left their children with sitters so they could go out and have fun. In my line of work, I've had conferences with parents I knew were alcoholics and drug users. They were prostitutes and had their children stay home to take care of the younger siblings while they went "out," yet here **I** was with cancer. *God, what are you doing, and how much longer are you going to punish me? My whole life has been one great struggle after another, and just when I thought things were finally going great, you give me cancer!* I was numb and in shock.

Cancer is a despicable killer, silently growing inside, many times causing destruction without you even knowing what is going on until it is too late. It changes one's perspective about everything. I was surrounded by love and had the support of my family and people I knew, but I was completely alone. No one could help. I was young. I had a career I loved. My marriage was great. Yet, I was dying.

I had two lymph nodes involved, so there was a chance that the cancerous cells might have gone through my system and were just waiting to flare up somewhere else. As a result, the plan was to have a lumpectomy and then chemotherapy and finally radiation.

I should have been grateful that I didn't lose my breast. After all, there are some women who have lost both, but the only thing I could think of was how unfair this whole thing was to me. Although I only had a scar, I still didn't understand why **I** was chosen to have to go through this ordeal in the first place.

My husband didn't understand me at all. He kept asking why I was so upset about a scar that no one could even see. He kept saying that I was acting like the scar was the end of the world instead of the idea that I had cancer. He said that if I had been a stripper, then he could have seen why I was so upset. He just didn't get it. I guess it takes being a woman to understand why this was so traumatic to me. After all, women spend so much money on breast augmentations for a reason. I wondered how he would feel if it had been one of his "jewels" that they were cutting on. Would he still take it so lightly? I knew I should have been grateful that it really was not an issue to him, but secretly, I was irritated that he wasn't sensitive to how I felt.

I cried daily because I just wanted my life back. Just a plain, normal, healthy life. *Why can't I have problems like other people? I wouldn't mind having my car repossessed or my electricity cut off. Family problems? Marital problems? Well, okay, fine. I'll take that, but this? Why couldn't I just have the everyday, mundane problems that other people have?*

Why did mine have to be a matter of life and death? …Well, just death, because everybody knows that with cancer comes death.

People say that we will all die one day, and yes, that's true. The problem is people assume that they will live a full life, see their children successful, happy, and with children of their own. People think they will grow old together with their spouses after living out their dream. All of these assumptions are encompassed in the statement, "We will all die one day." What about those who haven't lived a full life and still have things to accomplish? What about the people who still have dreams deep inside of them that have not yet come alive? What about their children who are still young babies? What about <u>those</u> people? That statement seems hollow, and cold. I wonder what they would say if <u>they</u> were the ones facing death! That statement is so easy to say when it's about someone else.

One night before falling asleep, I promised God that if He would just let me wake up and be in someone else's shoes or just let this whole thing be a dream, I would not complain about wanting a bigger house. I would stop thinking about how nice it would be if we had a second home down south or contemplate about the best way to invest money. I would stop trying to figure out how we would be able to retire earlier. Yes, I would get my priorities in order and simply enjoy what I had, because I now knew how precious life, health, and family are. I told God He could count on me to keep my promise to Him if He would just reverse this curse on my life. I woke up the next morning with the same life. Nothing at all had changed. God didn't hear my prayers…once again. I wondered if He ever did!

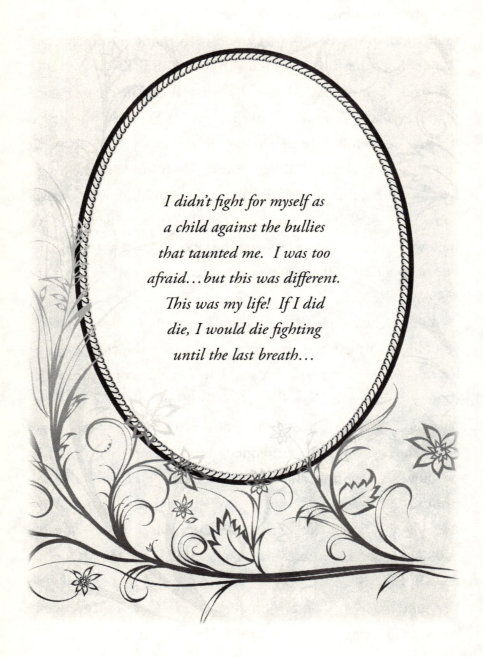

*I didn't fight for myself as
a child against the bullies
that taunted me. I was too
afraid…but this was different.
This was my life! If I did
die, I would die fighting
until the last breath…*

Chapter Two

My Journey Through Chemo

I wanted to start chemo as soon as I could. I couldn't stand the thought that every breath I took and everything I ate was feeding the very thing that was trying to destroy me. Imagine that. My own body had turned on itself, and the only thing that might be able to save it was poison. I now had to take poison to kill the disease that was trying to kill me.

Driving to the doctor's office for treatment was like going to a funeral. I prayed for strength the whole way to the doctor's office, and when I walked in for my first treatment, I was nervous, frightened, and sick with worry. My husband sat quietly and was in deep thought. I was still in shock over how my life was turning out. I still couldn't believe it. I kept waiting to wake up from this nightmare, but it kept going on and on and on. I was determined that I would not simply sit back and let this thing take me out without a fight. I didn't fight for myself as a child. I let the bullies run right over me, but not this time. I was going into the ring to fight with all I had. If I died, I would die fighting. Even if I lost the battle, my family would know I was not a quitter.

The infusion wasn't bad after they were finally able to find a vein. My veins have always been very small. Drawing blood was always an ordeal, but considering everything I was facing, that was the least of my concerns. My husband kept pacing back and forth with a look of defeat on his face, so I tried to encourage him by saying that God had everything under control. I told him that this whole ordeal was for a purpose and that in the end, God would get the victory out of it. I told him that the devil was not in charge, but God was allowing it for a greater good. Everything I said seemed like it fell on deaf ears. He continued to pace and contemplate. He tried to smile, but the smile didn't reach his eyes. I knew he wasn't listening to me at all. I smiled and hugged him and told him to quit worrying so much, but inside my heart, I cried for him, myself, and the life that no longer existed.

After the one-hour infusion, my husband took me to Jack's Deli for a corned beef sandwich, since I hadn't eaten all morning. Fear will do that to you. I've always wanted to lose weight, but certainly not like this. People kept telling me to eat to keep up my strength, but who can have an appetite when you are dying? God hadn't heard any of my prayers. If He had, I wouldn't be here, and they were talking about eating.

Anyway, I got the corned beef and practically inhaled it. I hadn't realized just how hungry I was until I started eating. I had to breathe a sigh of relief because I had been expecting the worst with the chemo, and it wasn't bad at all. The medicine they had given me to control the nausea had worked. It didn't hurt, and I didn't feel any adverse reaction to it. Well, at least something was going right. We got home, I thanked God for an easy day, and I put on my pajamas and climbed into bed, trying to think of something else, anything else except that dreaded "C" word. I started to pray again…when suddenly, I got this feeling in the pit of my stomach.

I put my hand over my mouth and ran downstairs to the bathroom, fell on my knees, and that's where I was for the next thirty minutes, face in the toilet. It seemed like everything I had eaten in the past three days was coming up. I couldn't stop, I couldn't catch my breath, I couldn't even get up off my knees. I heard my daughter in her bedroom crying, but I couldn't even stop or get off the floor to comfort her. With my face in the toilet, I cried too. The nausea medicine didn't work. I hated my life.

I took the next week off from work, and during that time, I was either drugged up or running to the bathroom. I'd wake up in the mornings, take my meds, eat a cracker, and throw it up fifteen minutes later. I got so tired of running downstairs that I finally just took my pillow and lay down on the bathroom floor by the toilet and closed my eyes for a bit to rest until the next wave came. At one point, I was throwing up so violently that it came through my nose as well, and I prayed that God would not let me die this way. I didn't want my daughter to come home from school and find me dead on the floor from suffocating on my vomit. Obviously, that never happened. Well, at least He heard that prayer.

I had lost all ability to taste anything at all. Everything tasted bland, so I ate jalapeño peppers with everything just so

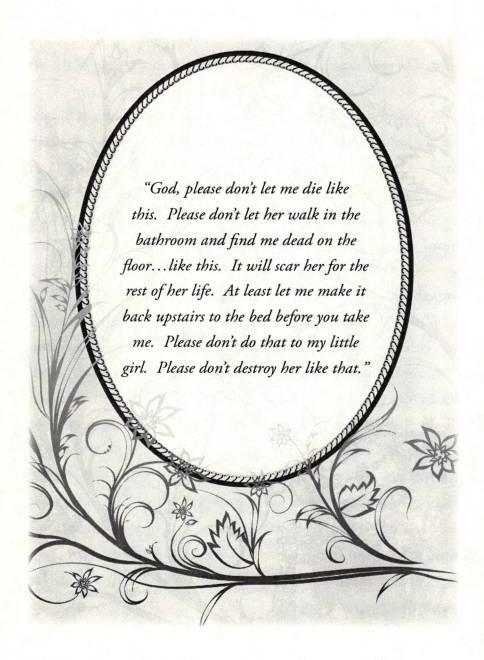

"God, please don't let me die like this. Please don't let her walk in the bathroom and find me dead on the floor…like this. It will scar her for the rest of her life. At least let me make it back upstairs to the bed before you take me. Please don't do that to my little girl. Please don't destroy her like that."

I could taste something. My smell, however, was very sensitive. Everything I smelled caused me to throw up. Food, lotion, shampoo, flowers. Anything with a scent forced me into the bathroom.

I was given meds after meds after meds in an attempt to control the nausea, but the only thing that did was keep me drugged up. Once, my daughter called to check on me, and I answered the phone. I didn't recognize who she was and told her she had the wrong number and hung up. I can only imagine how that must have cut into her heart. How sad that a mother didn't even recognize her own daughter's voice.

As each day came and went, my nausea became better, and by that Sunday, I felt well enough to go back to work, so I had a time frame now. Chemo on Friday, take the next week off, and go back to work the following week and repeat the process the next month. Great. So this was going to be my life for the next six months. Perfect.

About three weeks later, I was back at school and just getting back into the swing of things and getting my strength back when I sat down and ran my fingers through my long, black hair. Thick strands of hair came out in my hand. My hand was still in midair, my mouth fell open, my shoulders slumped forward, and I felt tears rolling down my cheeks. When was this going to end? Yes, I knew I would lose my hair. I was prepared for it, until it happened. Nothing can prepare a woman for this. A scar you can hide. The hellish week after chemo you can push back in your mind. The big, black cloud that follows you every second of every day sometimes you can push out of your mind…laughing at a joke, or comforting a friend in *her* time of need, or helping a student understand a concept. But how does a woman deal with no hair?

You are constantly reminded of it. Wearing scarves every day, all day. The time it takes having to match the color of the scarves with the outfit. I spent so much money at the fabric store so I could make my own scarves, but what alternative did I have? No, if I had to wear scarves, then I was going to do it up right! I wasn't going to wear a wig. That was simply out of the question. Wearing a wig looks natural until you want to scratch your head and can't, and you are always worrying about whether it is still on straight. It's one thing to shave your hair out of desire or to make a statement, but quite another thing to see wads of it in your hand because it is helping to keep you alive. I spent my lunch crying over my hair. Life had been so cruel to me. My life was a curse.

I had so many mental struggles I was dealing with. I knew it was all in my mind, however, that did not negate how I felt. I also knew what I saw. I gained so much weight in the short time after I started chemo that I went from a size ten to a size sixteen! None of my clothes would fit. I had spend time over the summers designing and sewing a lot of my outfits, and now none of them would even fit. I felt old, ugly, deformed, and useless.

I knew I would have to tell my students what was happening because I would be wearing scarves for the next six to nine months, but what would I say? I will never forget the support I received from my students. They all rallied around me and said it was a good thing that I was losing my hair. That just meant that the chemo was working. God had surrounded me with little angels daily to remind me that it was all right and this too would pass.

I finished my six months of chemo and breathed a sigh of relief. The blood work came back good, and the scans showed no new sites. My doctor said that if I made it out of the five-year window, there was a good chance that we had caught it in time. If it comes back, it's usually within that five-year period, so I made sure I went for my yearly checkup. Finally, my life was given back to me, and <u>this</u> time, things would be different. I became more aware of my eating habits. No chocolates, cookies, and the other goodies I loved to eat. That was hard, but every time I felt like complaining, I'd think about the ordeal of chemo, and I got over it. I even started juicing. I was going to do everything in my power never to have to see cancer enter my life again.

It took a while for us to get back into the swing of things, but slowly, things got back on track. I was certainly more aware of God and His awesome mercy towards me and my family. I made every effort to go to church every Sunday. Although I was never one to cuss when angry, I made it a point to watch my language and do all the things that "good Christians" do.

Chapter Three

God, Why Again?

My life was back on track, and I had a new appreciation for life. I knew that God had watched over me, and I was more aware of His presence in my life than before. However, every headache, flu bug, or bruise I got, my husband wanted to rush me to the hospital. That was a big problem between us. I couldn't tell him when I was sick because he always thought the worst and wanted a battery of tests run when only an aspirin was needed. Because I would refuse to go to the hospital when he wanted to take me, he felt like I was being careless with my health, and we became very frustrated with each other. Although it had been almost five years since cancer had ripped through our lives, it still held my husband hostage. I knew it would take time for him to work through it, and it was now my turn to be patient with him.

One March, I starting coughing. I hadn't gotten a flu shot, so now I was going to pay for it. I took all the medications I could get my hands on, but nothing worked. After about a month of continuous hacking, all day and all night, I developed a sharp pain in my left side. I could not stand straight, and it was painful simply to walk. Walking up and down stairs was like torture because it took so much effort just to move. It was difficult for me to even bend over to brush my teeth. I couldn't laugh, sneeze, or even breathe in deeply. Driving was an ordeal, especially backing up—and my car is a five-speed, so shifting gears made me cringe.

I finally went to the doctor, who had an x-ray done. Sure enough, I had cracked a rib from all the coughing. It seems that I didn't have a cold at all, but an allergy. I was taking medicine for a cold, not for allergies. How stupid is that? But then again, the only allergy I'd ever had was to cut grass—in the summer. This was March, and snow was still on the ground. Why would I take allergy medicine?

I was given the correct type of meds and told it would take six to nine weeks for my ribs to start healing, but in the meantime, I needed to take it easy. Sure enough, the meds worked, and I stopped coughing, but after nine weeks, I was still in pain. I was tired of limping, and walking around with a cracked rib was not wise when working in a middle school. I went back to the doctor, who decided to do a complete bone scan to see what was going on, and that's when they found them: three spots on my spine.

God to the rescue! It's interesting, but now I was beginning to see God in a different light. He had spared my life time and time again. Maybe He wasn't out to get me. Maybe there was a purpose for everything. Could it be that He was allowing me to go through this for a reason? The way I saw it was, had it not been for the allergies which I had never had, I would not have started coughing. Had it not been for the coughing, I wouldn't have cracked my rib, and there would not have been a need for the scan which caused us to find the spots on my spine when we did. It's funny. Although I knew God had stepped in just in time, I was still a little irritated that He was allowing me to go through this again.

Back to the oncologist we went. A bone biopsy was done, and it was cancer…again. I had almost made it out of the five-year window. It was four and a half years. So close, and yet so far. I was doomed. My life was over, and I was dying. This wasn't a scare like last time. This was for real. It had come back. I was in total shock. It was Y2000—so much for a new millennium.

There we were, back at my oncologist's office again. My husband kicked into survival mode and asked all the pertinent questions, and I just sat, numb and in shock. As my husband and I sat in the chairs across from my doctor, I heard her say that since the disease had gone to another area, it was now considered stage four, and there was no cure. The only thing they could do was give me treatment, which was to start in two weeks, and focus on quality of life. Oh, yeah, I was also told by a nurse to get my affairs in order. I couldn't even cry, because my mind simply shut down. My husband helped me up, and we walked stoically down the hall. Once we were out of sight of the other patients, he grabbed me and held me so tightly I couldn't breathe. I tried to look up at him to tell him how sorry I was for messing up his life, but he pushed my head into his chest and just held me. I think maybe he had tears in his eyes, and he didn't want me to see it.   My husband is such a strong man, but this even shook him.

The drive home was a very quiet one.   Both of us were lost in our own thoughts.   It pretty much stayed that way for several days.   I continued to go to work, but I was functioning more like a zombie—just going through the motions.

I couldn't understand what I had done to God that was so bad that He would allow this to happen to me.   As I thought back over my life, I was all right as a person.   I'm not saying that I was perfect.   I had my flaws, like everyone else.   I was still dealing with the utter rage and immense unforgiveness I felt for the two men that murdered my mother over fifteen years ago.   The raw hatred I felt for them was still fresh, but I had that tucked safely away.   I couldn't forgive them.   I was angry because the death penalty was not an option in that state, and they got to live.   I knew what I felt was wrong, but I didn't care. She was my mother, and I wanted them dead.   There, I said it. I wanted them to die the same way they killed her, but with a sweet little twist.   I wanted, just before their life left them, but while they were still conscious, to know that the "gift" was from me, the daughter of the woman they murdered.   Oh, how that thought brought me such sweet pleasure.

I could have had "something" done to both men.   A few people came to me to offer their "services." I didn't seek them out. I will not say the thought never crossed my mind.   Not only did

I think of it, I meditated on it. Yes, I admit it. I thought long and hard about "it." It was so tempting and quite easy. It's all about knowing the right people who have nothing to lose, and having a little bit of money. I had both. I actually thought of it as a good investment. Every time, however, I decided to set it in motion, I kept hearing that scripture that says, "Vengeance is mine," or I'd remember when my mother took me to church as a child and learning about Jesus. So many good thoughts would seep back into my mind to counter the "other" thoughts. After months and months of contemplation, I decided not to do it. No, I was not afraid. I had already decided that I would never spend one day in a prison, no matter what I had to do, and I was prepared to do "it" if necessary. After all, what did I have to lose? But I did the right thing and let the justice system handle it. It was extremely difficult for me to walk away from the prospect, but I did, because it was the right thing to do.

Yes, they were both sentenced to life in prison, but because of a problem with the way the search warrant was written, one man got life with parole and the other life without parole. Daddy had died from a freak accident two years earlier. I'm glad Daddy had already been gone when this happened to Mama. This would have tormented him to his death. Mama was dead by their hands, and I got a death sentence handed down by my own body. I hadn't even done anything and yet, I was in my own prison. Oh, the dark, barren places I have had to travel through on this path called life.

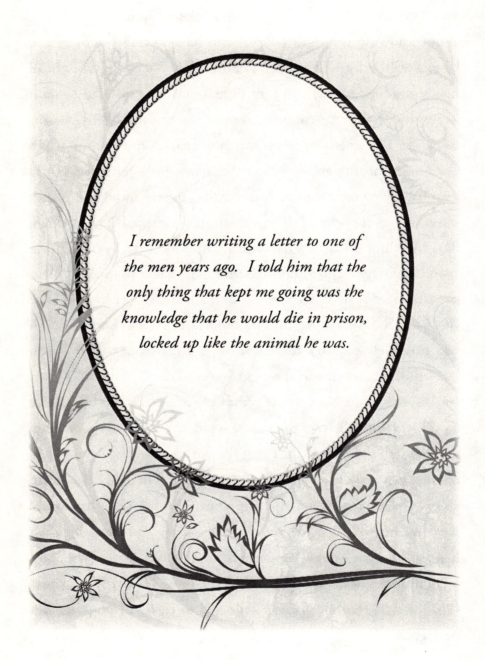

I remember writing a letter to one of the men years ago. I told him that the only thing that kept me going was the knowledge that he would die in prison, locked up like the animal he was.

I had all of those emotions tucked safely away from the world, so I knew that I was far from the perfect person: but why couldn't God see that I had done the right thing in the end? I didn't do it. I didn't avenge my mother's death, so why must I suffer through this death walk…again?

Everybody's life seemed better than mine. I was jealous of everybody—even the squirrels. I'd look at my friends and wonder what had they done that was so good that caused them to be able to escape my curse. I'd even look at the prostitutes, the drug addicts, and gamblers and think how lucky they were. They had an addiction that could be helped, but they had their health. How could a prostitute be in better health than me? The most I could get was "quality of life" until the treatments stopped working and the cancer finished eating me up alive.

Things that seemed so major to me were now insignificant: The latest fashion trends I just <u>had</u> to keep up with. The newest diets I tried just to be able to squeeze into a size four pant or the various products I desperately tried to simply lighten my freckles. Yes, vanity does go before a fall!

So many days, I'd just drive to work, sit in the parking lot, watch my colleagues walk into the building, and wonder what it must be like to have a life like theirs. Yes, they had their own problems, as everyone does, but it's all in the way you look at things. No matter how I looked at things, I had a "sucky" life and was now dying. It had been so long since life was "good" for me—good in the sense that I had no major problems on the surface. Yes, we all have "character-building" things we can work on, but that would come in time. Time was quickly ticking away from me. Pre-cancer was so long ago. I couldn't even remember what if felt like to laugh without cancer.

Chapter Four

The Start of My New Beginning

My heart ached for my husband. Although I had my own pain, I could see it in his eyes and hear it in his voice. This strong, feisty man looked haggard. He had withdrawn within himself so much that there was only a shell left, and it was all because of me. All of the dreams and plans we had were gone. Poof! Just like that. Everything, completely gone. One day we were talking about buying some property in Florida for a second home for when we retired, and the next day…death. I felt despair and complete hopelessness. Where was God? When was He going to step in and stop this madness? It seemed like one moment He was all present, my hero, working things out, and the next, He was nowhere to be found. He had turned His face from me.

I loved my husband so much, and I knew what I had to do. I had been thinking about this for a while. Sometimes, the right thing to do is the hardest, but I had no choice in the matter. Cancer had taken all choices away from me. I didn't even feel like a woman anymore. I couldn't even remember what it was like to feel like a woman. My skin still felt leathery from the chemo and radiation from the initial time. I hated even standing beside other women, because it reminded me of how I wasn't one anymore.

When I went to the grocery store and a woman stood in line in front of me, I would let a man in front of me so I wouldn't have to stand beside the woman. Simply standing beside her made me feel even more of a man. When my husband and I held hands and walked down the street together, I felt sorry for him because he was walking beside another man—me. I walked with my head down and shoulders slumped forward. Who wants to look at someone so ugly? I am younger than my husband, and someone once asked me if he was my son. Yes. That was confirmation to me. I was an ugly nothing, and the taunts from my childhood resurfaced…

The kids would laugh at my long, wavy hair and my eyes, my mother's eyes. They told me how ugly I was. They called me horrible names and made fun of me for being bi-racial. From first grade to twelfth grade, the girls called me ugly and "slow." They were right. I was. All I could think about was the scars… scar was on my breast. Another scar was under my arm from where they had to take lymph nodes to test. Scar on my mind, scar on my heart; Scarred in my spirit. Oh, how I hated myself.

My husband and I had such a wonderful and passionate life before cancer. Even though it had been almost five years since cancer, I still couldn't see myself as whole again. Gone were the pretty, frilly nighties and the silky teddies. Terry-cloth house shoes or just plain white socks replaced the fur covered sexy slippers. Satin bed linens-gone. Playful, dual languages were not spoken anymore. Gone were the looks that said a thousand words that only we understood. Gone were the giggles and the secret whispers.

In their place were silence and distance. Not from him, but from me. Entered in downcast, sad eyes and a harshness in my voice I couldn't control, sweats and a t-shirt clothed me in the bed. I didn't even want the cute sweats. The more raggedy they were, the more comfortable I felt.

My husband would buy me beautiful things from Victoria's Secret, but I never wore them. I didn't want him to see how ugly I really was. For some strange reason, he still thought I was beautiful! I couldn't let him see how wrong he was. I was a defect, full of scars. He deserved so much more than this, and now God was allowing it to start all over again. I took a deep breath, walked upstairs, and told my husband I wanted a divorce. God was destroying me piece by piece, but I would not allow my husband to be destroyed alongside of me. I kept thinking to myself, if you love something, then you must set it free.

I'll never forget the look on his face when I said that word, *divorce*. It looked like someone had kicked him in the stomach with steel boots. His whole face seemed to simply drop. He said he couldn't believe I would even think of that, but he was all I could think about. I was dying, so why should I take him down with me? He still had a life. What kind of life would he have watching me die a slow death? No. I couldn't do that to him. I spent most of my life alone. It seemed only right that I spend my

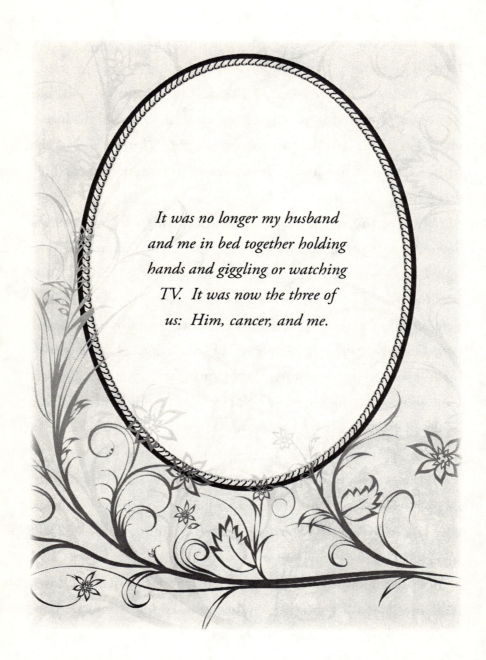

It was no longer my husband
and me in bed together holding
hands and giggling or watching
TV. It was now the three of
us: Him, cancer, and me.

end alone.   Instead of him agreeing with me or even thinking about divorce, he was devastated that I would even think of it.

My husband didn't understand the beautiful gift I was trying to give him. I was giving him his freedom. No strings attached. It was a gift from my broken, dying heart. Yes, it killed me to say the words, but he deserved so much more than me. I remember once, during one of my surgeries, because there were no more cots or even a chair available, my husband slept on the cold, hard floor beside my hospital bed. He used his jacket as a pillow. How could I deny this loving man his life? He was such a loyal, honorable man. I *had* to give it back to him!

My husband told me he wouldn't give me a divorce because he loved me - no matter what. He said an illness couldn't change how he felt for me, and that he wasn't a machine who could cut it on and off like that.   He refused to even consider it…

It's amazing how God orchestrated our relationship from the very beginning. I wasn't looking for a husband, or even "husband material." It just happened. Now I understand why it is critical to wait for God to send you a mate, because He will send you the one who can stand the storms when they come up in your lives. I smile when I think of our first meeting. He wasn't my type and I thought he was arrogant, (which was and still is such a turn-off to me) but look as us now. That same man that "wasn't my type" was actually my soul mate, and God had already planned our "meeting."

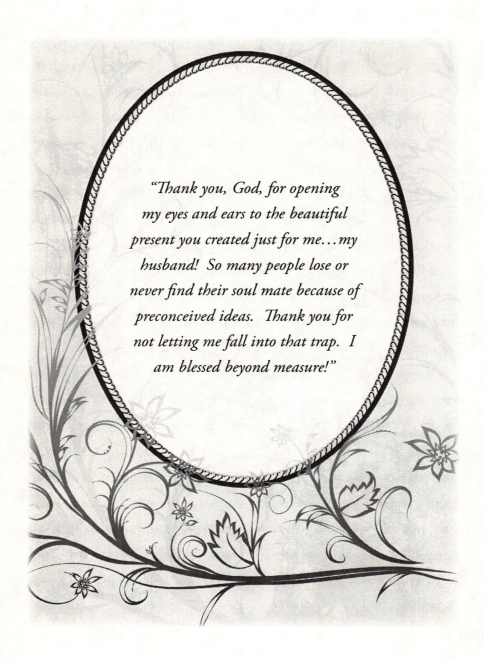

"Thank you, God, for opening my eyes and ears to the beautiful present you created just for me…my husband! So many people lose or never find their soul mate because of preconceived ideas. Thank you for not letting me fall into that trap. I am blessed beyond measure!"

Well, I was told I should start thinking about getting my affairs in order. How do you do that? Whom do you call? *Do I pick out a casket first, or find a place to be buried? Do I write a will? Do I pick out what poem I want to be read? What do you do?* I had no idea what to do, and my heart was heavy because I still couldn't believe that this was how it was all going to end. I decided that I had to quit feeling sorry for myself and get down to business. I had to do this for my husband. The least I could do was get things in order so he wouldn't have to try to make any decisions after I was gone. It would have already been done for him. Yet, every time I tried to pick up the phone to inquire about the process, I would hear, "It's not your time" or I'd simply hear the word, *"premature."* I tried over the course of one week to make the call, but each time, I'd hear something in my spirit that made me stop.

I even started writing letters to my family to be opened at various times in their lives, but I could never find the strength to complete the letters. Something just kept telling me, "Not yet."

In frustration, I decided that I would focus my attention on my spiritual life, because simply doing nothing was driving me crazy. I would make sure that when I left this earth, I would end up in the arms of my Lord. I knew that once I had that part of my life situated, then everything else would come together and I would be able to make the necessary arrangements.

I began to earnestly pray and seek God. I mean <u>really</u> seek His face. I wanted what the Bible talked about in the Book of Acts. I knew I had to get "filled with the Holy Ghost with evidence of speaking in tongues" (Acts 2:24). I was on a new mission. I was beginning to feel revived, because now I was doing something to fight instead of sitting back and watching it being done to me. According to the Bible, this was a gift that anyone could have if they wanted it. That Tuesday, I went to prayer service with a purpose, and that was to get what the Bible said was mine. Since I was going to die so early, I would die with His spirit in me. The last words I intended to speak after saying my goodbyes to my family was His heavenly language. I wanted to be ushered into His kingdom speaking a language that no one could understand but Him.

At church, after singing a few worship songs, I went to the altar and began to pray. There was so much I had to be sorry for. I prayed for my family, and my sisters and brother. I prayed for Mama and Daddy, who were long gone. I prayed that my husband would find a nice woman to be with, but that I would always be his real love. I prayed that the hatred and unforgiveness I had for the two men who killed my mother would be gone by the time I died so I could be clean when I stood before God. I began to praise and worship Him, and my heart filled with adoration for Him. I forgot all about the cancer but only focused on my love for Him, and then it happened…

I was on a hill, kneeling before the cross. I was crying, and I could taste the grains of sand and dirt in my mouth, mingled with my tears. I looked up and had to bend my head back all the way to see Him. He was on the cross, but it was so high, and I could barely make out the outline of His feet. My heart broke as I imagined the pain He must be going through, and as I opened my mouth to tell

Him how much I loved Him and how sorry I was that this happened to Him, I began speaking words that I had never heard of or spoken before.

He did just as He said He would do. He blessed me with the precious gift of the Holy Ghost, and He did it in such a beautiful and memorable way. He took me back to His earthly ending to start my spiritual beginning.

Now I was ready to face chemo again. My first treatment was planned for that following week. I had a plan, and I had power. I had God's spirit working in me. I was ready. I wasn't unrealistic. I knew that it would still be hard and I would still hate what I was going through, but I *knew* it was going to be all right. Before each treatment, I anointed myself with oil and prayed over my body. I would even put a little oil on my finger and touch the IV and pray that the medicine would do just what it was designed to do. I took my Bible and read scriptures on healing as the poison slowly dripped into my veins in its attempt to keep me alive.

This chemo wasn't as bad as the first one, but it was much longer. I went in at 8:00 a.m. and was hooked to an IV until 4:40 p.m. It was such a long day. Advancements had been made on the chemo to make it more tolerable, so I didn't have the nausea, although I did lose my hair again. You would think that after going through it once, I would be used to it. Wrong. It had been about five years ago that I lost my hair, and here we were again. Once again, I cried my eyes out. I wondered, how much more was I to endure? Although I had the Holy Ghost inside of me, I was still tired of going through this roller-coaster ride. Please understand that the Holy Ghost does not excuse you from life's trials, but it does give you the grace and strength to stand until victory comes. Now there was this small ember of fire burning deep down within the innermost core of me. The doctor's report did not change, but how I looked at it did. My body was tired, but my spirit was strong.

I had always had this fight in me, but this was a different kind of battle. It's hard to explain. It's more like a spiritual fight had always been going on, but now I was privy to it. Knowledge is power. God says, "My people are destroyed for lack of knowledge" (Hos. 4:6). I had the knowledge now. New fight, new rules. When you are fighting in the physical realm, you fight with feelings and what you see. As a matter of fact, the only way to get the advantage is to see from every angle. You use all of your senses. Not so when it is a spiritual battle. Here, we wrestle "against principalities, against powers, against the rulers of the darkness of this world, against spiritual wickedness in high places" (Eph. 6:12). In this kind of fight, you must arm yourself with the ***word of God***. It's not about what you see, but what you know God's Word says. Feelings and senses have no place in this arena. It's above that. Satan doesn't care about your feelings, tears, pain, or anything else. He is a spiritual being. He does *not* want you to use the word of God against him. This is how the battle is won: "Speak the word daily."

Think about the three times Satan came to tempt Jesus in the wilderness (Matt. 4:1-11). Each time, Jesus counterattacked Satan by speaking the word of God to him, and finally, "the devil leaveth him" (v. 11). You've got to believe this and know that it works. Even in my dreams, the enemy was after me, and the word worked. I once had a dream that *I was held hostage in this room. There were two men sitting in the outer room playing cards with the TV on. Their job was to keep me locked up until the general came.*

One man came in the room and let me out of the cage and attempted to take me downstairs, but before he could, someone called for him, and he let go. He intended to come back for me, so he didn't lock me up again. As he left the room, I sneaked out of the building and escaped. As I began to run, I started calling on the name of Jesus, and each time I did, I began to fly. I flew over many houses, and as I looked down, I could see the men running outside, screaming at me. I flew to the rooftop of one house and hid behind the chimney, and then everything was quiet. As I peeped around the chimney, I saw long, pointed fingers gripping the edge of the roof. The general could fly too and had found me. It pulled itself up, and I could see its horrid face. It was covered in black hair, but not like a dog or cat. Its hair was more like a boar's, coarse and sharp. It had long, pointed ears with big, oversized eyes. Its eyes were filled with complete, pure evil. It snarled at me, and I could see razor-sharp fangs growing out. I quickly grabbed it by the face and kept flinging it back and forth on top of the roof. Each time I flung it, I called on the name of Jesus, and each time, it got smaller and smaller, until finally, it was just putty in my hand. I flung it against the chimney so hard that the jerking of it woke me up and I found myself gasping for breath in the middle of the bed.

I truly believe that God was telling me through my dreams that the battle had already been won in the spirit. I now had to walk it out in the physical realm.

Chapter Five

The Death Angel in Paradise

I finished my nine months of treatment on June 29, 2001, and I was ready for a break. My daughter and I went to Hawaii for one month to visit my sisters, who were living there. Because of work, my husband couldn't go, but I desperately needed something different, so on July 10th, my daughter and I left without him.

Spending time with my sisters was wonderful. We talked about the "good ol' days," went shopping, and went to church. We did some sight-seeing, but not much, because I was still recuperating from the chemo. Walking along the beach and smelling the salt air as the sun beat down on my back was so relaxing. It's funny, but all I could think of was the vitamins in the sun that would help my hair grow faster.

My sisters and I talked so much about the Lord. They were at a different place in their walk with Him than I was. They kept telling me I needed to develop a relationship with God. I had no idea what they were talking about. I didn't want to tell them this, but I secretly thought they had gone off the deep end! They were taking this "God" thing just a little too far. I mean, I knew

God. I went to church, and I prayed. But come on, what kind of relationship can you have with a Spirit? They did suggest that I should begin journal-writing about my experiences while there, which did sound sane and reasonable. They seemed to believe that something awesome was going to happen while I was there. My sisters were so optimistic, and I loved them for it.

I remember going to church service about two weeks later, and the Holy Ghost fell, and everyone was in the spirit. Some people were dancing before the Lord, others were weeping at the altar, some were running around the sanctuary, and others were lying prostrate on the floor before Him. The atmosphere was electric, and His presence was felt in a mighty and powerful way.

In the middle of this, a lady came to me and said, "I have been arguing with God about this all evening. I didn't want to come over here, since we don't even know each other at all, but I have to obey Him. He said to tell you that you would be healed." Tears filled my eyes as I hugged this stranger who had obeyed God and delivered a life-changing message to me. I began to dance before Him in the spirit. Yes, He <u>had </u>heard my prayers. He <u>would</u> spare my life. Without a doubt, I knew there was a God and He was a Healer. My sisters were right. They had sensed in the spirit that something big was going to happen, and it did. I now knew God had heard my prayers!

My time on this paradise island flew by. I didn't want to leave. I had a connection with God while on that island, but I knew it was time to go back and get ready for the new school year. I had lesson plans and tests to rewrite, activities to make up, and field trips to plan out. I had purchased a lot of things and decided to box them up to send home. This way, I didn't have to worry about carrying them myself. So, Tuesday evening, I began packing for our Friday trip back home. I had just finished taping up the last box and was so proud of myself that I was able to get everything in only three big boxes. Tomorrow, I would send them off.

After saying goodnight to everyone, I prayed before bed, but this prayer was strange. I thanked God for such a beautiful time with my sisters and asked that He would give us a safe trip home in the coming days. I then said, "God, out there is someone who has all these plans for tomorrow they want to accomplish. But they don't realize that the death angel is in the room with them and that the bed sheets they pull up over them tonight will be their wrapping sheets. I just ask that You have Your hands over them and their family and give them the strength to go through what they will have to face." I then prayed again that He would give us a safe trip home, and I got into bed, pulled the sheets over me, and went to sleep.

Miyako, my daughter, tells me that in the middle of the night, she began hearing a strange noise that frightened her. She kept tossing and turning, trying to ignore it, but the noises wouldn't stop. Finally, she got out of bed to ask me to go see what the noise was. To her horror, it was me making the noises. According to her, I was on my back and my back was arched upwards, my mouth was open, and my eyes were rolled back. She screamed and ran to the back of the apartment to my sister's room to tell her what was going on. My sister assured her that it was only

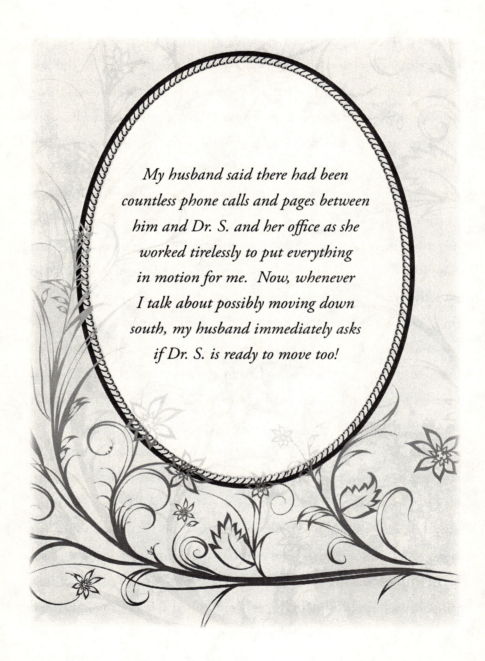

My husband said there had been
countless phone calls and pages between
him and Dr. S. and her office as she
worked tirelessly to put everything
in motion for me. Now, whenever
I talk about possibly moving down
south, my husband immediately asks
if Dr. S. is ready to move too!

a dream and that she should go back to bed. My daughter was frantic at this time, and finally, my sister got out of bed to prove to her that all was well, and that's when she found me. Instantly, she rolled me on my side and ran to the bedroom to make calls. While she was on the phone, I threw up; still unaware of what was going on. My sister made three phone calls. She called the pastors of her church to start a prayer chain, as well as the EMS.

By the time the EMS arrived, I was unconscious and non-responsive. I was rushed to the hospital and assessed. My sisters were told that I was in critical condition and would not survive the night. According to the scans performed upon my arrival, they could see something on my brain, but because of my history with cancer, they didn't know what they were dealing with. Also, the location of the problem made it difficult to treat. In essence, they told my sisters to get the family together to take the first plane to the island, although it was doubtful if anyone would make it in time. The doctors said there was no time to waste. My one sister asked, "Isn't there anything you can do?" to which the doctor replied, "Miss, you don't understand the seriousness of this. Your sister will not make it off of this island alive. I'm sorry."

My sisters called my husband, who in turn called my oncologist. Dr. S. told him to get me back home any way possible: "She needs to be back here." At this point, I was in and out of consciousness and unaware of the seriousness of my situation. I vaguely remember speaking to my husband, who was practically hysterical by this time. He asked if I thought I was

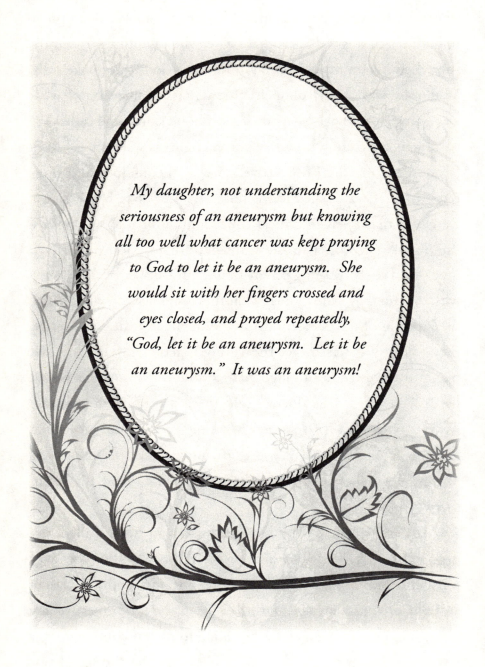

My daughter, not understanding the seriousness of an aneurysm but knowing all too well what cancer was kept praying to God to let it be an aneurysm. She would sit with her fingers crossed and eyes closed, and prayed repeatedly, "God, let it be an aneurysm. Let it be an aneurysm." It was an aneurysm!

able to travel home and said he would fly to the island to fly back with me. I told him that was silly and a waste of money, that I was perfectly capable of flying back without him. (I still did not know how serious I was.) Because of my condition, the airlines did not want me on board, so I had to sign papers releasing the airlines of responsibility for me. The hospital did not want to release me, and again, I had to sign papers for them to release me. My sister traveled with us, but what I didn't know was that this was the only way the hospital would release me. My sister was told that I would probably die before the plane landed, and my daughter, who was only eleven years old, should not be left alone with me when I passed away.

When I was released, we went from the hospital straight to the airport. We left with only the clothes we wore from the hospital. My other sister would have to pack up our things and send them to us later, but for now, we were fighting against time. The last flight off of the island that night would be leaving in three hours, and we had just enough time to make it. The flight back home was long. There was a lay-over in California and Chicago. I was in slight pain, but I had been given a good dose of morphine, so it wasn't that bad. I was more worried about my sister because she would be missing work because of me and I didn't understand what the big deal was.

When we finally arrived back home, my husband met us at the gate and ran towards us. I still didn't understand why he was so upset, because no one had yet told me how dire my circumstances were. I told him I wanted to go home first and rest, but he ignored me and took me straight to the hospital, where there was a team of doctors waiting for me to arrive. Dr. S. had set the whole thing up. There was a flurry of activity as I was registered and given a room.

Once situated, I was given several more scans, and finally, I was able to rest. I had been poked and prodded and asked countless and pointless questions, like my name and the year and the name of the president. I just wanted to sleep. Finally, the scans were back. The doctors could see something on my brain, but blood was obscuring the view. Whatever it was had started to bleed, but for some unknown reason, it had simply stopped. As a result, they were not able to get a clear view of the area, so they would have to wait five to seven days for the blood to be reabsorbed back into my system before rescanning. Their hands were tied. They couldn't treat me until they knew what they were dealing with, yet time was working against me. The problem was that the doctors in Hawaii said that every day I delayed some type of treatment, my chance of survival would lower by fifteen percent. Added to that was the fact that, upon arriving at the hospital in Hawaii, it was said that I had less than a fifty-percent probability of survival, so the chances did not look good for me at all. During that week, I only remember my husband feeding me and sleeping.

Another scan was given six days later, and finally, a good picture could be seen. No, it was not cancer. I had an aneurysm, and surgery was scheduled for the next morning. My husband was given the best- and worst-case scenarios. Worst case was that I would die on the table. The best-case scenario was that I would make it through the surgery, but would probably suffer a stroke, and I'd be paralyzed. That morning, before the surgery, my husband stood beside me as we held hands and he prayed for my life.

The next thing I remember is being in bed after the surgery and my husband telling me I had made it. I was only in the hospital three days after brain surgery before being released. Everyone was amazed at how quickly I had recovered. Although we had excellent insurance, my doctors told my husband that I didn't need to be there with sick people; that I should be at home, where I could recuperate even faster. It seems that one of the criteria they use to determine mental stability is whether one can tell or laugh at a joke. Well, one question they asked me was who the last US President was. I won't say what name I gave, but it will be interesting to see if the name I spoke jokingly turns out to be our next President. We shall see.

Nonetheless, I was weak and slept for about one week before actually trying to stay up. I remember taking a bath one night, but then I couldn't get out of the tub. I sat there and cried for about fifteen minutes while trying to lift myself out of the tub before calling my husband. I didn't want him to see me like this, scarred up and too weak to even get myself out of the tub. Yes, now there was one more scar added to my body: one that went from my right temple to my left temple from the surgery. My hair was finally growing back in from the chemo, but now I had a long scar across the front top of my head, so I still had to wear a scarf. I cried again.

I was home two weeks before I started physical therapy. My legs were weak, and although I was given a walker to help me to move around, I refused to use it. I instead used the wall and objects around to help me walk. My husband would get angry with me for not using the walker, but I just couldn't see myself having to use that thing just to get around. Looking back on it now, I believe that was because so many things that had happened to me were out of my control and this was something that I could control, so I exercised it.

The first home visit from the therapist was difficult. I couldn't even bend down to pick up a piece of paper or touch my toes, but he taught me exercises to do until his next visit later that week. I couldn't believe how much strength I had lost during this ordeal, so I exercised as instructed. By the fourth visit, two weeks later, this is what the therapist said to me: "Ma'am, I make my money according to the number of patients I see. That is how I make my livelihood. The more patients I have, the more money I make, but I can't even justify coming back here anymore. You have made remarkable improvements in just two weeks. I wish all of my patients could respond as quickly as you have. What is your secret?" I told him that I serve a God that can do anything. He looked at his chart and shook his head and said, "You just had brain surgery, and you are already at home and walking around without help." He signed me off of his caseload and left my house, still shaking his head.

I went back to the neurologist six weeks later, and when I walked in and gave my name, the nurse standing on the other side of the office looked up when she heard my name, and pulled me to the side. She went on and on about how well I looked, and then she said how lucky I was, because people in my situation usually don't make it out alive. She said the staff felt so sad for us the night before the surgery as they checked on me and saw my family surrounding me. It seems that no one expected me to make it through, and when they wheeled me out of surgery and I was still alive, they were all shocked, but still expected the worst. And to see me alive and doing so well was unbelievable. I told her that God has always watched over me and it was Him that brought me out safely. She said she didn't know who I served, but the angels certainly were watching over me.

If she only knew. I was very much aware of what God had done for me, again. This was the sixth time that He had commanded the angel of death to stand back. Six times, going all the way back to when my mother carried me in her womb, death has tried to snatch me. I wasn't even supposed to be born. Each time, the Master of creation said "No," and every time, death had to obey.

This ordeal really changed me. I saw God's hand all over my circumstances. He spared me. I should have died. According to everyone in the medical field, I'm not supposed to be here, but God said, *"No."* He loves me and had not forgotten me. Although I have had to walk through this valley, and it seemed like I was alone, He was always there.

Something inside me started to change. I wanted to please Him. I wanted to be what He wanted me to be. Change happens from the inside out, and it's something that is not always seen on the outside. It's like planting a seed in the ground. You water it, even though you can't see what is happening under the earth, and then one day, a tiny sprout shoots out and is seen. I had to change, and it started on the inside with a decision to do so. My biggest battle was the hatred for the two men who murdered Mom. I thought I had dealt with it. I mean, I didn't wish death on them anymore, so as far as I was concerned, I had done my part—but God said, "Not so."

I knew this was going to be a major battle for me—even bigger than the one I was fighting in my body. The Bible says we are to love our brethren as we love ourselves. *How do I love the people who completely destroyed my world as I knew it? How do I forgive the monsters that invaded my life, snatched my mother from me, practically took my sanity away, and left me a shell of a person? How?*

I knew prayer was the key, but I didn't want to pray for them, so I had a long talk with God. I explained to Him that I didn't want to pray for them, but I was just doing it to please Him. I wanted God to understand that I was not a fake. My prayers for these two men were not sincere, but done strictly out of obedience, and so it started. Each morning, as I talked to God, I grudgingly said, "And bless D and R." That's all I could say, and I almost choked on those words, but I had already told God that it wouldn't be sincere, so....

I did this every day for many, many months. Then one morning, as I was praying, it slipped out, and I asked God to show up in their lives so they might know Him. I literally stopped praying to think about what had come out of my mouth. Shocking, but I decided that even they should know who He was. So, this was my prayer for several more months.

One morning, as I was praying, I saw a steel cage and thought how absolutely horrific it must be to spend your life locked up in a cage, and I thought of D. and R. I tried to imagine a typical day in their lives, and I began to ask God to make a way so that they would find Him—I mean, really get to know Him and His love. I was surprised that I was slowly beginning to pray heartfelt prayers for them. No, I still didn't feel this brotherly love for them, nor did I want to. I told God I would pray for them, and I did. <u>He</u> would have to do the rest, but I wasn't going to help. I would just continue to pray the way I had been, and the rest was up to God.

Chapter Six

Climbing Up the Rough Side of the Mountain

Things in my life were on an incline. No more chemo; my strength was coming back, as well as my hair. I could finally breathe. 2001 had been a nightmare, but I was still here. I kept up with my monthly visits to my oncologist, and my personal life was good. I had the usual scan, which I took every six months to track the disease in my bones, and I did this like clockwork.

On one of my visits in 2004, when Dr. S. walked in, she wasn't cheerful as usual. My scans were not good. There were three spots on my liver. The disease had progressed to an internal organ. This was very serious now, because an internal organ was under attack. Bone is very dense, so if the disease had to spread, spreading to bone is a good thing, but it hadn't stayed there. This was not good at all.

We began discussing possible types of treatment…again. Surprisingly, I didn't cry this time. Maybe I was just tired of going through the same thing, maybe I became so used to it, or maybe I knew that I had recently had another death walk and God had

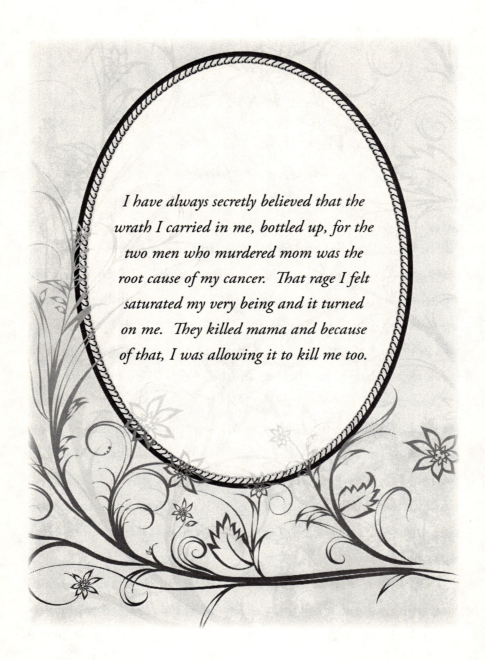

I have always secretly believed that the wrath I carried in me, bottled up, for the two men who murdered mom was the root cause of my cancer. That rage I felt saturated my very being and it turned on me. They killed mama and because of that, I was allowing it to kill me too.

brought me out of it once before: He was with me then, and He would be with me now. Whatever the reason, I sat there and discussed the treatment and planning of it, just as I did my own lesson plans for school. Upon leaving, my doctor hugged me and said how sorry she was, and I just smiled and said, "Everything will work out the way it is supposed to, and I still thank God." She looked at me with a puzzled expression on her face, and I said God determines what happens and when. No one leaves this earth until God says it's time. Not even cancer has that much power. She smiled her big smile and said, "You are right, and you are amazing," and I replied, "No, God is amazing."

Driving home, I prayed and thanked God for all He had done for me and my family. I thanked Him for allowing us to find this new site when we did. I had just been given devastating news, and all I could do was thank Him for being God. It's ironic. My faith in God was growing, but I also saw myself growing more and more ugly. It's like the inside of me was blossoming but the outside of me was wilting. When I looked into the mirror, I saw such ugliness and deformity. I became so disgusted in myself, but what could I change?

I remember once I spent over $600.00 in one day purchasing cosmetics, thinking that would make me look better. Excitedly, I came home and made myself up with my new makeup, and my loving husband didn't notice a thing. I stood in front of him and asked him what he thought. He looked at me and said, "About what?" I gritted my teeth, smiled, and stuck my face out. He studied my face and had the nerve to ask me if I had new lipstick on. New lipstick! I just spent $689.00 on makeup, everything from the skin care treatment to the various eye color palettes to make me look pretty to him and the only thing he could pick out was *lipstick!* I could have thrown a chair at him because of all the money and effort I had put into making myself more appealing, and he didn't notice a thing. What I didn't realize is that what I saw in the mirror was not the same thing he saw. He still saw me. The same woman he had fallen in love with years ago. I saw cancer and the entire disgusting residue it left behind.

One weekend before I was to start my new treatment, I developed a sudden, sharp pain in my lower stomach. I suffered the whole weekend, thinking it was nerves or maybe something I ate, but I went to my doctor's office early Monday morning. A new scan was taken, and the results came back. I now had a kidney stone. So on top of everything else I was dealing with, I now had to deal with that. I was told to change my diet and try to get it to pass, because the pain would persist and only get sharper until the stone was passed. Easier said than done. *How do you pass a rock?* I thought. *If I drank a lot of water, it would force me to use the bathroom and that would be excruciating pain. If I didn't, this rock would continue to stay there causing pain as well.* Great. *I've heard about it from other people, and now I am living it. Just my luck!* I wanted to scream out and ask God what more could happen to me, but I was afraid I might find out.

I was at school two weeks later and got so sick I could barely stand. As I was standing in the library with some students, a pain hit me so hard in my lower stomach that I fell to my knees. I knew something was wrong, but was it the kidney stone or had cancer now spread to my stomach? The not knowing was driving me crazy on top of the pain I was experiencing. I somehow drove myself to the hospital, praying all the way. It was sheer determination and God's grace that I didn't pass out from the pain. I went to the oncology floor and as soon as the receptionist saw me, they took me right back. I had a temperature of 103 and was dehydrated. I was admitted instantly. It seems that I had developed an infection, so they gave me antibiotics through an IV and gave me saline for the dehydration. Somewhere, something happened, and my blood had become too diluted. Now, I needed a blood transfusion.

So, this is what my life had come down to: Mama's murder, cancer, reoccurrence, brain aneurysm, reoccurrence, kidney stone, and now a blood transfusion. Surprisingly enough, throughout this whole time I was in the hospital, I continued to trust in God and I kept thinking of the power in the blood of Jesus. I prayed that He would touch this "new" blood that I would have to get and cause it to restore me. I prayed that this "new" blood would somehow change me and that I would leave the hospital a different person. I was discharged three days later.

Upon coming home, my daughter told me that someone from the parole board had called me and I should return the call, which I did. Much to my surprise, one of the men who took Mama's life had died. He had had a heart attack. He was only in his forties, and it had happened at the same time that I was in the hospital. I had prayed and dreamed for this day, for his death, and now it had finally come. The man who murdered my mother was now dead, and it didn't happen by my hands. I had no blood on my hands. His blood did not cry out from the ground because of me, but surprisingly, I didn't want to celebrate. I actually felt sad. My heart was heavy.

After I hung up the phone, I cried for him and for his family. They had lost a son, and at one time, I'm sure he was an adorable little boy. For years, I thought of him as a demon from hell, but he still had a family who loved him. He was God's child who had simply listened to Satan for that one brief moment and it cost him his freedom, and my mother's life. I begged God to forgive him for taking Mama from us. I told God that we have all sinned, and that one sin is no larger than another. I pleaded with God to forgive him and said I had forgiven him for what he had done to me. I lay before God and petitioned for his soul. I prayed for his mother and father because no parent should ever have to bury their child. I prayed for mercy on his life and that he had found God before he died.

That very next day, I passed the kidney stone. I often wonder if the passing of that stone was a signal that my body was expelling the deep-seated unforgiveness and hatred I had held onto for so long. Just days earlier, I had prayed that the "new" blood I received through the transfusion would change me, and I found myself pleading to God to forgive the man who murdered my own mother. God had heard my prayer. I was changing. I kept the stone as a tangible reminder of a mountain that God removed from my path.

The following week, for the third time again, I started my treatment. I went through one treatment after another. We stayed with one until it stopped being effective, and then we moved on to something else. I took the treatments, but my faith in God was increasing. There was something on the inside of me that said, "It's not your time." I tried to look at things objectively, because I am a realist. *If this is my time to go, so be it.* I am not one of those people who believe in positive thinking or positive energy, because this is *not* faith. People often confuse positive thinking with faith. Faith is the realization that God can do all things. The more I prayed and read the Bible, the more I began to realize that God was bigger than this cancer and that God was using what was sent from hell to His glory. Yes, one day I will leave this earth, as all people will, but I was beginning to feel that it would not be now, and not by cancer.

Thank God that cancer research had come a long way and the drugs available didn't tie me to the toilet like the first time, so I was still able to continue to work and take treatments on Fridays. God blessed me with the strength to be able to bounce back and be at school by Monday, almost completely recovered. Unfortunately, I did lose my hair again. The third time of losing my hair due to chemo and yes, that made me cry. How silly is that? I didn't shed a tear when cancer was found on my liver, but I cried like a baby when my hair began coming out. I remembered the words of my students from '96 who said, "It's a good thing that your hair is coming out. It means that the chemo is working." You would never think that God speaks through children, but He will to get His message to you, so we must be careful not to dismiss the words of a child, for they can hold many truths.

I have always had dreams, but God began to give me dream after dream, and visions. In each of them, I was not sick. I began to read books on healing. Out of the blue, people I didn't even know would make small talk with me and talk about how they were diagnosed with cancer and given months to live and were healed. Once, I went into a local natural health food store to purchase vitamins, and the clerk began talking to me about this herb he was taking. He said he had been diagnosed with cancer years ago and was only given a few months to live, and he was healed, so he now takes this certain vitamin to keep his immune system up.

A lady at the church I was visiting shared her testimony with me, not knowing my situation. She talked about how she had cancer and the doctors could do no more, and she "turned it over to God." That was eleven years ago. Time and time again, I was hearing testimonies of cancer healings from complete strangers. The more I heard it, the more my faith was built up, and I began to believe that if He could do it for one, He could do it for me. After all, the Bible says, "God is no respecter of persons" (Acts 10:34), so…

After months and months of prayer, consecration, and studying, I had a major breakthrough. I realized that this thing called life was not about me and my wants and needs. It is about serving God and preparing ourselves, not for this world, which is temporal, but for what is to come—eternity. He knew us before He formed us. "Before I formed thee in the belly I knew thee" (Jer. 1:5), and He knows what we can take and what we can't. He is the thermostat in our furnace of affliction. This is why some people had an easier walk through cancer than I did, and there are some whose walk was much more difficult.

I used to be envious of people who would come to me for counsel because of a bad or questionable medical report. After my first bout with cancer, I became known as the poster child for cancer. I am a very private person, and God gave me the grace to walk through this without people even knowing it came back on me, so people would think nothing of talking openly about someone who had recently passed away or a bad result, not knowing I was going through it again myself. I would talk to them and encourage them as they poured out their hearts to me.

Many times, I would come home and put my needs aside and beg God for their health. I knew what was in store for them if the test results came back positive, and I asked Him for mercy on their behalf. It was as if I took these people in my hands and lifted them up over my head to heaven and asked God to reverse the bad report and send forth healing. There were times I fasted for others and their healing...and He heard the prayers. Sure enough, they would always come back thrilled about the good news. One time, the report came back wrong. Another time, it turned out to be benign. Yet another time, it was caught in time, and a simple lumpectomy was needed, and no chemo. Still another time, it turned out to be fibrosis. There were different people with different, but positive victories. They would hug me, and we would cry tears of joy together, but through all of the laughter and high-fives to God for their victory, some of my tears would be for me.

As happy as I was for them, my heart ached because I wanted to know when it would be my turn. I knew God could do it, but why wasn't He? When would it be my turn to laugh and cry because of a breakthrough? I saw the hand of God move in other people's lives around me, but His scepter never lowered towards me. I could never understand why He would deliver other people around me, but not me. If I didn't know God, I would have thought it was almost cruel how He would have me pray and fast for others and then I would have to stand there and watch them get blessed. It was always just within my grasp, yet out of my reach. But as this happened over and over again, I began to understand that He knew what I could handle. God was strengthening me. No, I was still fighting cancer, but I was also developing a relationship with Him—that thing my sisters had talked about in Hawaii.

I was learning how to praise Him in my trial. Slowly, I was depending more and more upon Him and less and less upon me. Let's face it—what I was doing wasn't working anyway, but that does not mean He is not able. I am reminded of the three men, Shadrach, Meshach, and Abednego, who were cast into the burning fiery furnace by King Nebuchadnezzar (Dan. 3:20). Their faith in God never wavered. They understood that God was

God, whether they were in the furnace or out. I was beginning to understand what they meant.

Does this mean I enjoyed it? Certainly not, but I will say that He was there with me through the whole ordeal. When I was at my wits' end, He would give me a dream or send a piece of mail telling me about a miracle service taking place in a state nearby. He always sent something or someone to encourage me when I was on a downward slope.

Once, my husband had come home from visiting a church, and he told me that at the end of the message, the pastor had said someone in the room had something to do with cancer. He said he didn't know who it was or what the detail of it was, but God was saying that He was working it out. Was it a coincidence that this pastor just happened to say this on the very same night my husband just happened to attend? No, I do not believe in coincidences, but my husband had a divine appointment to be at that church on that night to hear that comment. God knew what we needed to hear to hold on, and He set things in motion. Actually, He had set this thing in motion before we were even created, because He knew the walk I would have to take.

As I go back through time, back to my childhood, I can now understand why my life was so difficult. I know why I was so alienated and despised. The nights I cried myself to sleep, the days I was forced to run home from school, the times I stood in the background and watched everybody else laugh and have fun were to strengthen me. It is almost a parallel to my walk with cancer. Many times, I stood by and watched everyone laugh and enjoy life when I knew my life was slowly ebbing away. As a child, I learned how to play alone. As an adult, I sat in my car and cried because my walk through cancer was such a lonely one. He had been preparing me since I was a child for this death walk that I had to endure, because this was the first phase of what He has planned for me. "The steps of a good man are ordered by the Lord" (Ps. 37:23). I am simply amazed at how awesome God is and how He had ordered my steps from the beginning of my life. What as a child I once thought of as a curse now became a blessing for me. When people whispered about me and my prognosis, it didn't destroy me. I didn't shrivel up and run and hide. I was used to the whisperings. When I was alienated and taunted as a child, it taught me to keep on walking, so when cancer came to stop me, I just kept on walking and have continued to walk.

Chapter Seven

The Victory Through Him

In July 2007, my blood count jumped up to 507. Normal is between 0 and 30. Also, one of the spots on my liver had grown larger, so I had to begin a different type of chemo once again. Although I had been on various types of hormonal treatment since 2004, we now were back to the "hard stuff", but you know what? I did not shed one single tear. *I have wasted too many tears on this. I know what God said to me. I know what He showed me in my dreams and visions. No more. I'm done. Satan, I quit. No more will you cause me to stay up nights and worry and become depressed. I shall not put my life on hold. Cancer is* not *the ruler of my life, but my Lord, Jesus Christ is. I will not shed one more teardrop over this.* As a matter of fact, I began to praise Him, because whether I have cancer or not, He is still God. He still sits on the throne, and He is watchful and mindful of everything that happens to me, to you, and on His planet. Jesus said in Matt. 10:30, "But the very hairs of your head are all numbered." *He knows the number of hairs we have on our heads, so if He is going to allow this, so be it. I will walk through it like I have everything else my whole life. I have gained a*

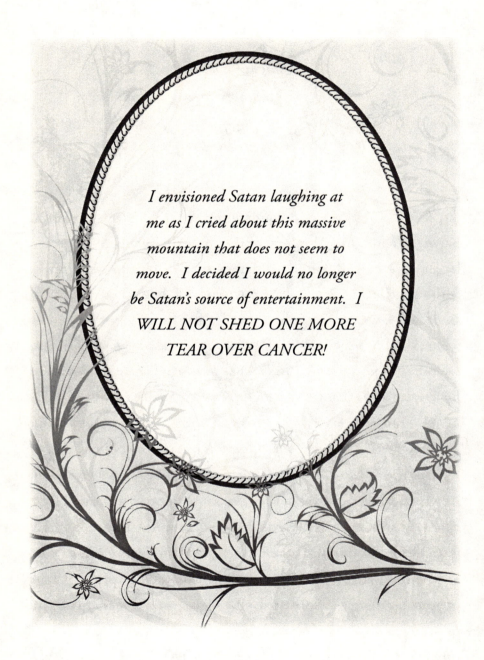

I envisioned Satan laughing at me as I cried about this massive mountain that does not seem to move. I decided I would no longer be Satan's source of entertainment. I WILL NOT SHED ONE MORE TEAR OVER CANCER!

deeper relationship with Him. I am hopelessly in love with Him, and every day is an adventure. I'm always wondering what will He show me or tell me today. What revelation will He open up to me?

One of the ways He speaks to us is in dreams, so whenever I had a dream, as soon as I woke up, I would write it down and begin to scrutinize it. And you know what? I was excited to hear what He had to say. Remember your very first love? Remember how you couldn't wait to hear his voice or what he had to say? Well, I was back to that time of my life, only better, and it was exciting. Sometimes I would just journal-write what I heard in the spirit, and it is amazing, the peace and level of understanding He will take you to if you will simply seek Him and listen.

In Is. 43:26, it says, "Put me in remembrance," and I did that faithfully. Each day, I prayed health over my body. Each morning, I would say, "With His stripes, I am healed in Jesus' name, and no weapon formed against me shall prosper." I took scripture and turned it into a prayer that was relevant for my situation. Each time before my doctor's visit for a treatment and before each office visit to get results from my scan, I would remind God of how He said He would heal me. Each time, the scans would show stability, and my doctor would rejoice.

In October 2007, I finally found a church that I could call home. The very first time I attended the church, the pastor prophesized over me and told me that there had been a premature death in my family. (My mother was killed when she was only forty-eight.) He said that there had also been an assignment for a premature death for my life, as well, but God said, "Not so."

(Cancer, the aneurysm, carbon monoxide poisoning, and other times I should have died that I didn't mention here.) He spoke things to me that no man could know unless He was hearing from the Almighty Himself. I visited this church for a very short time before joining. Since that time, I have grown in my walk with God. Both he and his wife, also a pastor, encourage me, and they pull out of me what God has placed in me that I can't see myself—but they see.

This book is because of my pastor, an anointed man of God who is also an apostle. He prophesied and said I was a writer. People had always told me I should write a book, but I never took them seriously. My pastor spoke that to me, and I began to think about it seriously. This book is birthed out of his leadership. Because of their ministry, I found myself so focused on God that my desire is to only please Him, not to remind Him of what He said He would do for me.

At the end of November, I had an appointment to discuss my test results. This was usually the time I'd remind God of His promises and pray for my healing, but this time, I forgot. Can you believe it? I forgot to pray for myself. As I was driving to the doctor's office, I was busy singing praises to Him and thinking about how I could serve Him more. I had fallen in love with Him and not His gifts. I didn't matter. My health didn't matter. I just wanted to please Him. I just wanted Him. I walked into the office with my mind still on Him, and Dr. S. walked in. She said she was pleased with the scans. There were two places they had been concerned about, but those had since cleared up.

Everything else was stable, and one spot on my liver was even getting smaller. She looked at my blood count and began to smile bigger. My count had gone from 507 in July to 56.

It has been eleven years since cancer stormed into my life, seven years since I was told to get my affairs in order, and four years since the cancer invaded my liver. King David talked about walking in the valley of the shadow of death (Ps. 23:4): "Yea, though I walk through the valley of the shadow of death, I will fear no evil." I have literally walked along that path <u>several</u> times. It is a dark and lonely place. Although I had my family by my side every step of the way, it was still a long and lonesome walk. There are some things that you will go through in life where you cannot take your family with you. It is a walk that you must take alone, but rest assured, you are not alone, for you will meet God on the path. He is there, waiting for you to reach out to Him. Remember though, you are only walking through. You will not take up residence here, but it is a path some of us have had to walk through to reach our next level in God.

Yes, it has been a struggle. I have had to claw my way up from the pit, but as long as you continue forward, you will make progress. The first step is always the hardest, but it is necessary, for "Faith without works is dead" (James 2:20). You must step out on something that you don't see with your natural eye, and it will seem unnatural and scary, but He will be there, smiling, with outstretched arms, because you had the faith to step out.

I have had one form of treatment after another throughout these eleven years, and my situation has changed in one way or another, but the only thing that has <u>never</u> changed was God's word to me. God has been faithful to His word to me. Sadly, there have been people I met after my diagnosis that are no longer here, and yes, at times, my faith was shaken, but I know what He told <u>me</u> one day in 2000. Sometimes, all you will have is a word that the Lord spoke to you years ago. Hold on to that word. No matter what you see or hear. Hold on to the word of the Lord.

My husband and I were sitting on the couch watching TV and out of the blue, my husband asked, "Do you think this thing will take you out?" Immediately, God whispered in my ear, "This sickness is not unto death" (John 11:4), and He has stood by His word. The medical records did not line up with what He said. My body screamed a different message. I looked in the kitchen and saw one medicine bottle after another that spoke opposition to what He said, but you have to decide whose report you will believe. Will you believe the report of the doctor or the Master Physician? Yes, cancer came to kill me. It is a dreadful destroyer sent to wreak havoc on my family, my body, my mental state, and my finances. However, because of cancer, I have a story to tell that I pray will help others find their way to God, as I have. Because of cancer, I know that He is a Healer. Because of cancer, I have found out more about myself than I ever would have, and I was even able to put to rest the demons from my childhood.

Unbeknownst to me, unforgiveness had a life of its own and was eating away at me little by little, and I didn't even realize it. It was as if I had it locked up in a cage, buried deep within, where no one knew it even existed: but like a Pandora's box, cancer pried it open and everything came pouring out until I was freed of its venomous grip. Cancer forced me to face the **stronghold** that unforgiveness had on me and finally kill it with the forgiveness sent from God. Because of cancer, I have found the best pastors there ever was. Because of cancer, I know my husband loves me unconditionally. I have pushed him away in an attempt to spare him, and he still wants me. I have scars that are hidden to the outside world, but he sees them all, both inside and outside the body, and he still finds me beautiful. He still desires me. Had it not been for the cancer, I would have never known these truths, these nuggets of gold buried deep inside of me and my husband.

Chapter Eight

Cancer, I Salute You

If you are reading this book, it is because cancer has touched either your life or someone dear to you. Yes, I know all of the emotions you are going through. I have had them myself. I remember lying in bed at three o'clock in the morning while my husband slept, screaming unheard cries in my mind. The countless times I'd wake up to a tear-soaked pillow from where I had been crying even in my sleep. I remember celebrating a birthday and wondering if it would be my last time. There were so many potential last times for me. Last time going on a family vacation? Last time barbequing on the Fourth? Last time going to a work function? It was like everything I did, I wondered if it would be my last time.

I'd look at myself in the mirror and literally despise what I saw. I didn't see me, but I saw this thing that was trying to kill me. My body was trying to kill itself, and there was nothing I could do about it but continue to breathe—but in breathing, I was giving it life as well. I forced myself to carry on like normal because I didn't want to burden my family any more than was necessary. The way

I handled this would determine the atmosphere in my home, and it was hard enough for them to sit by and watch knowing there was nothing they could do. I couldn't show them how tired and broken I was, so I learned how to pretend…at first.

Yes, I carried all the spirits of fear, doubt, and anger around for a very long time. They were my best friends…I thought…but in actuality, it was all a set-up to break my spirit. It was sent "priority" from the very pits of hell. If your spirit is broken, there is no will to fight or survive, and then you become easy prey. Remember, the scripture talks about how "the devil as a roaring lion, walketh about, seeking whom he may devour" (1 Pet. 5:8). If he is seeking, that means he's looking for the weak one. Not weak in body, but weak in the spirit.

The Bible says, "God hath dealt to every man the measure of faith" (Rom. 12:3). This means you were already created with some faith in you, but it is up to you to exercise it. Stand on what was given to you. You have everything to gain! Don't just give up. I don't care if cancer does run in your family and every other member in your family… That doesn't mean your story has to end up the same way. You can be the one that breaks the generational curse on your family. So what if they said it was in the last stages? They told me that too, but here I am, twelve years later. God is the author and finisher of all things. He has the last say. Not the doctors.

I almost lost myself because all I could think of was my cancer and death, but it is a spirit sent from the pits of hell to stunt your growth and belief in the One who can set you free; the One who can give life. It is the enemy who has come to kill, steal, and destroy, but the Lord came to give us life. He simply wants us to believe Him more than we believe the enemy. No, I am not saying not to listen to the counsel of your doctor. That would not be using wisdom. I did everything my doctor told me to do, but I knew this was really a battle that was being fought in the spiritual realm manifesting in the physical realm.

Back in 2000, one afternoon after it had came back in my spine, as I was lying on the bed praying, I saw two huge, warring angels. One was dressed in a white robe with gold trim along the front collar and around the hem of the sleeves. There was also gold thread sewn within the garment. It stood probably eight feet tall and held a sword that had what looked like a mother-of-pearl handle. It too, was trimmed in gold. Standing across from it was another angel, dressed completely in black, equally beautiful and gigantic. I stood there as they began to fight. The ground shook violently as these magnificent beings moved to and fro, and I fell to the ground because of it. The sound of blade hitting blade was deafening, and as I looked, light hit the blade of the angel in white and blinded me. I held up my arms to cover my face, and then I understood everything. (It was as if the light illuminated truth to me!) As I shielded my eyes, I stood up and whispered to myself, *They are fighting over me. They are fighting over my life.* As soon as I spoke those words, I heard, "IT IS DONE." Suddenly, my eyes opened, and I was back on my bed.

I know some people may think I am crazy or that I was hallucinating, but this is what I saw. *I knew then and I know now* *that this **was** and **is** a spiritual battle being fought in the physical realm.*

Did this make my fight easier? No, it did not. I still had to go through chemo and everything that comes with that, but something changed in me after that. I can't explain it, but I knew that there was more going on around me than what I could see with my natural eyes.

You must develop a "warrior" spirit within you. There is a real entity trying to take your life. You cannot simply sit down and allow it to take you over. You must build up your arsenal and begin by filling your spirit-man with words of life and faith. Get a journal and begin reading about the people that Jesus healed. Come on. What do you have to lose? All you are going to do otherwise is sit, worry, and talk yourself into a depression, and what does that accomplish? Write the occurrences down and study them. Meditate on scriptures of healing and faith. Immerse yourself in words of life. Begin a prayer life. No, you do *not* have to kneel down and recite a formal prayer. It's hard to concentrate on Him when your knees hurt. I believe the posture in your heart is more important than the position of your body for prayer. Sit on the bed and just talk to Him, or lie prostrate on the floor before Him. Talk to Him while you are driving or working. Cry out to Him. He will listen. That's all He's ever wanted you to do. Cry out to Him earnestly and wait quietly, and He will whisper back to you, and then write down what He says. (Don't forget to date it.) You are beginning a *relationship* with Him. Then ask Him to come into your heart. It will turn into a beautiful love song that no one can sing or hear but you and Him—an unending love affair that no man can match.

As for my scars, they are still there, but I now see them as battle scars. They remind me of God's love and mercy for me. They are a visible sign that I was in a war with death and I came out victorious, through God. The bloodier the battle, the more wounds are had, but I have lived to tell about my battle scars, and I do so through this book.

So, here's to you, cancer. I salute you. You have taken many prisoners in the past, but the Blood of Jesus is against you here. Had it not been for you, I would still be playing church. I would be doing all the seemingly "right" things that people do when they think they are serving God—things like going to church every Sunday and Bible study on Thursdays. Perhaps I would hold some type of position at church, or maybe even teach Sunday school, but I would never have known the priceless relationship there is to have with the King of Kings and Lord of Lords. I would not know the peace I have when I go into my prayer closet and spend quality time with Him. I know when I pray, He hears me. I would not know what it feels like to get completely lost in Him and come back to yourself with power and no feeling of fear. After all, He has not given us the spirit of fear. I would have missed out on all that I have now.

Cancer, once upon a time, I used to cry because of you. I'd cry myself to sleep and even cried in my sleep. I cried at birthdays and holidays. I wanted to be somebody else, anybody else, but as I stand before Almighty God, I say that I would not trade my life for anyone else's in this world. I am blessed beyond measure. I have an anointing and relationship with God that cannot be purchased, but only comes through trials and walking through the furnace of affliction. The same people I used to envy, I now think of how much is missing in their lives.

Cancer, you actually pushed me to Him. You thought I would curse God, but instead, you forced me to run to Him. He had been watching over me and calling me with open arms all along. I just never paid any attention to Him until you came into my life. You came to kill me, but you actually saved my life. You are my enemy, and you came to destroy me, but I now stand on top of you and proclaim, "To God be the glory for all He has done for me, and I praise His Holy name." And I heard the Lord say...

"Sit thou on my right hand, till I make thine
enemies thy footstool" (Mark 12:36).

To You,

In the precious name of Jesus, whose I am and whom I serve, that at the name of Jesus every knee shall bow and every tongue shall confess that Jesus Christ is Lord. Father God, I plead the blood of Jesus over everyone who reads this book and that they may find You within the pages written here. I speak that the words written here will change lives and cause people to look to You for healing, strength, deliverance, and peace of mind. Matthew 16:19 says, "Whatsoever thou shalt bind on earth shall be bound in heaven, and whatsoever thou shalt loose on earth shall be loosed in heaven," so I bind every cancerous rogue cell in their bodies that does not line up and function according to Your Word, and I loose complete healing and restoration in the precious Name of Jesus.

Father, Isaiah 53:5 says, "and with His stripes we are healed," and I take You at Your word, so I speak healing in the bodies, in the minds, and in the families of everyone who reads this book. You are a Healer and a Deliverer, and I praise Your holy name. I thank you in advance for the healings and the testimonies that will come because of Your touch. Cleanse us and have Your way in our lives as You change us to become more like You. We praise You and thank You while we are in this battle, because You will make a way out for us through Your healing touch. This I pray in the Mighty Name of Jesus. Amen.

Chapter Nine

Practical Tips for the Ladies

1. Take a deep breath and understand that although you are in a life-threatening war, it does not mean that you have already lost. The doctor's report is not the last report. *God's report* is. If He can raise Lazarus from the dead, and He did, He can certainly take care of some out-of-control cells.

2. Be practical. Make adjustments in your life, and be prepared to make even more.

3. Reserve your strength. Allow others to help. This does not mean you are weak or giving up. Fight strategically, and save your strength for chemo and the days following.

4. When you do cook, prepare double portions and freeze them for later. You may not have an appetite or taste buds, but it's easier to take out something and warm it up than to start from scratch—especially when you will be irritated about the whole situation anyway.

5. If you are going to wear a wig, buy one before *all* your hair is gone. This way, you can get a better color match. Take it to your own stylist and have her cut it, but buy the two-sided

tape and tape it on before going. This way, the length will be correct. Also, keep in mind the fit. Once all you hair is gone, the wig will fit a little larger.

6. You might want to get bangs cut in. You will probably lose your eyebrows as well, and this way, the bangs will take attention off your eyebrows.

7. Before you go home, get a good eyebrow pencil and start using it. You want to be familiar with using the pencil and the natural shape of your brows, so drawing them in will not be so difficult. You know, there are some women who shave off all their eyebrows so they can draw in a different shape.

8. You might want to think about wearing your wig occasionally before "D-day" to get used to seeing yourself in one. It will seem a little strange at first, but you are still a beautiful woman. Hair does not define a woman. You are strong and you are awesome. Put your hair on, lift your head up, and "work it."

9. If you are choosing to wear scarves instead, start off by buying the basic colors first. Look in your closet and pay attention to the colors you have more of. You may want to go to a fabric store and buy fabric and make your own scarves. This way, you have control over the color and print. Making scarves is simple. It's nothing more than a huge rectangle. Have fun with wrapping them is stylish ways.

10. Start studying the Bible. Get all the scriptures on healing and health. Put each one on an index card, and tape them in various places in your house. When the enemy starts

whispering to you, speak the word back to him, like Jesus did.

11. Construct a prayer just for you. In other words, find scriptures about healing and include them in your prayer. Do not pray the problem. Pray the solution. Your prayers should always be positive and include God's promises to you about health.

12. Start a prayer journal. As you pray, write down what God speaks to you. It may be an audible voice, or something you simply "hear" in the spirit. It might be in a dream or a vision. Either way, it should be written down with the date and time. Trust me, as your walk with Him gets closer, you will want to refer back to previous things He has told you.

13. Separate yourself from people who are not speaking life to you. The enemy will use anyone to get your eyes off of God. Don't make it easy for him.

14. Ladies, if your husband buys you something pretty and frilly, don't do what I did and pack it away. He's trying to tell you he still finds you sexy and that he has eyes only for you. Remember, he is feeling helpless and lost, and this is his way of showing you he loves you and cares.

15. It's all right to be a little selfish. You've got to focus on you and your health right now. However, keep in mind that although you're going through the fight, your husband is sitting by wanting and needing to feel like he is doing something to help. Try to include him and fight this battle together, not separately. Remember, united you stand. Divided you fall.

Chapter Ten

Practical Tips for the Men

1. If your wife or loved one is going through this, it is important for you to follow her lead. You may want to take the lead here, but remember that it is her that is going through it and she is still trying to find her way. One day she may be happy and the next day in tears. Part of it is hormonal, and part of it is her coming to grips with her new situation.

2. Find a time during the day or evening where you can both sit down and read the Bible together. You can find scriptures and stories of healings that took place and discuss them. Try to help her build up her faith. You both need to know that this is not an automatic death sentence.

3. Help out around the house. She will probably feel bad because she is not able to do those things she is used to doing, but if you help out, she will not focus on it.

4. Surprise her with gifts occasionally. She may feel unloved—not because of you, but remember, the hormones are off. It doesn't have to be extravagant. A little card or a hand-written

love note hidden under the covers would be perfect. We like things like that.

5. Filling up the tank with gas is great. She will have so much on her mind that one less thing to do is a present. Especially if you don't tell her and she gets in the car and see it on "full"… which is what happened to me just this morning (smile).

6. Please, please don't try to be Superman. This affects you as well. It's your life, too. Share your thoughts and fears with her. Don't try to spare her and cut her out. She will feel even more alone. Yes, we women like strong men, but we love strong men who can cry sometimes. That shows his strength and tenderness, and you need her as much as she needs you.

7. Reassure her that she is still beautiful. This disease can play a serious mind game on a person. Continue to remind her that she is still every bit the woman now that she always was before…and show her.

8. Include her in things, and let her decide what she wants to do. You will want to exclude her so she can rest, but that may come across like you are planning your life as if she's gone already.

9. Be prepared for change…in *all* areas of your life. She is fighting for her life, and her priorities will change. Try to be understanding and patient, but above all, communicate with her. She needs to know what you think and how you feel.

10. This is very important. Begin right away with a routine of prayer. Hold hands and pray together, and you speak healing and health over her. Again, find scriptures to include in your

prayer, and don't pray the problem, but the solution. It doesn't have to be long. Even if it's five minutes, do it. Prayer does make a difference.

Final Thoughts

You will have your good days and your bad days. One moment you will feel encouraged and strong in your spirit and the next you will collapse in tears. That's all right. You didn't let God down for feeling this way. You are human. Don't forget that right before Jesus went to the cross, He prayed, *"O my Father, if it be possible, let this cup pass from me: nevertheless not as I will, but as thou wilt"* (Matt. 26:39). You may even go for a follow up visit and your doctor will say that nothing has changed. Possibly your cancer has even progressed, but do not panic. A DELAY IS NOT A DENIAL!

When this happens, simply wipe your eyes, say a prayer or read a scripture. A close friend of mine suggested that I get the Bible on audio to listen to when I wasn't up to reading. She was so right. Even when I fell asleep or didn't want to read, my spirit was hearing the word of God. The point is to strengthen yourself by immersing yourself in the Word of God.

My husband is constantly telling our daughter, it's not how you start that counts but how you finish that matters.   My prayer for you and for me is that we finish our course as strong as humanly possible and that He will look down upon us with a smile and say, Well done my good and faithful servant.   Well done!

I have gone through too much and I have come too far to turn back.

Though he slay me, yet will I trust in him (Job 13:15)!

God Bless You!

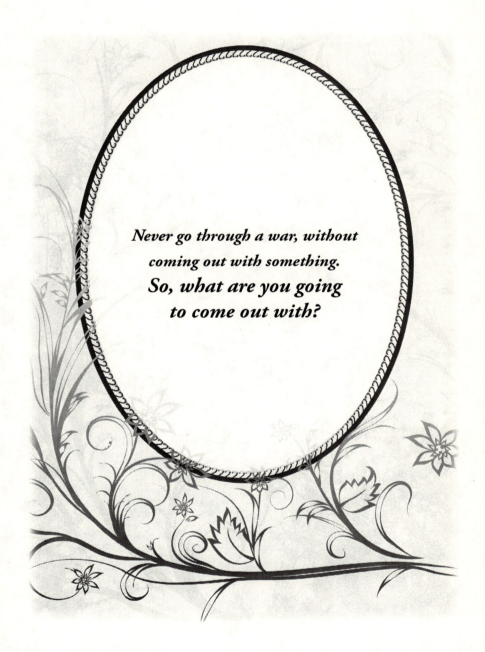

Never go through a war, without
coming out with something.
So, what are you going
to come out with?

LaVergne, TN USA
02 February 2010
171743LV00003B/54/P